DIY

Homemade Alcohol-based Hand Sanitizer

With Anti-bacterial, Anti-Viral, Anti-Fungal and Anti-Microbial Essential oils Recipes (19 Recipes)

By April .K. Brown

i

Copyright

All Rights Reserved. Contents in this book may not be copied in any way or by means without written consent of the publisher, with the exclusion of brief excerpt in critical reviews and articles.

April .K. Brown© 2020

Disclaimer

This book is projected to be a general guide, to raise consciousness, and to aid people to make knowledgeable decisions in the context of their circumstance.

The author takes no responsibility for any damage or injury be it personal or monetary, as a result of the use or abuse of the information in this book. If you have any doubts or worries after reading this book, do well to speak to a qualified person before further actions.

Table of Contents

Chapter 1

Introduction

Hand sanitizers defined

Hand sanitizer, sometimes called hand antiseptic, hand rub is a liquid, gel, or foam applied to the hands to get rid of or decreases common pathogens in them.

Hand sanitizers are a type of antimicrobial agent that, when applied on the hands permanently inactivate or kill a wide range of microorganisms like fungi, viruses, and bacteria.

Most hand sanitizers are hazardous if ingested because they are made of toxic chemicals, mainly alcohol, as their active ingredient.

According to the CDC, alcohol-based hand sanitizer that meets the alcohol volume (at least 60%) requirements rapidly decreases the number of microbes present on your hands. It also helps you avoid falling sick and spreading germs to others.

Note that even the best alcohol-based hand sanitizer has some shortcoming and do not eliminate all types of germs.

Hand sanitizer is recommended when soap and water are absent for hand washing.

Hand sanitizers may not work well for all settings, especially when the hands are visibly dirty or greasy.

Hand washing with soap and water is generally preferred because hand washing decreases the amounts of all types of chemical and germs and on hands, only use hand sanitizer in the absence of soap and water.

For a hand sanitizer to be effective against pathogens, it must have a final alcohol concentration of at least 60%, at most 95%.

How to use hand sanitizer

First: Apply or spray the sanitizer on the palm of one hand

Second: Put your hand together and rub it thoroughly.

Third: As you rub, cover the whole surface of your hands and fingers.

Fourth: Rub until your hands are dry or rub for 30 to 60 seconds continuously. It takes hand sanitizer at least 60 seconds or more to kill most germs.

What germs can hand sanitizer kill?

Alcohol-based hand sanitizer don't get rid of all types of germs such as norovirus (stomach bug), Clostridium difficile (diarrhea) and some parasites

<u>Advantages of alcohol-based hand sanitizer:</u>

Hand sanitizers are suitable, handy, and easy to use and require less time than hand washing.

Alcohol-based hand sanitizer acts quickly in killing microorganisms on hands.

It reduces the spread of rotavirus, adenovirus and rhinovirus present in the hands.

Hand Sanitizer can easily be accessed than sink; it saves you the stress of looking for a sink when in a hurry.

Hand sanitizer is a handy, on-the-go way to help prevent the spread of germs when soap and water aren't available.

Although alcohol-based hand sanitizers can be useful in getting rid of germs, health authorities still endorse hand washing at any time to keep your hands free of pathogens.

Chapter 2

Materials and Basic ingredients needed

- <u>Tools</u>

1 mixing bowl

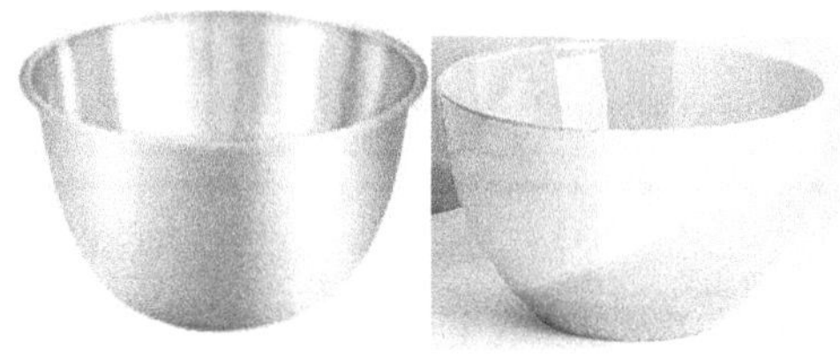

1 mixing utensil

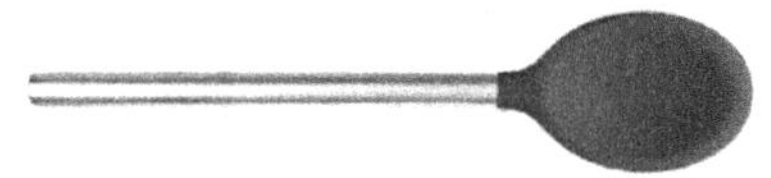

Clean funnel

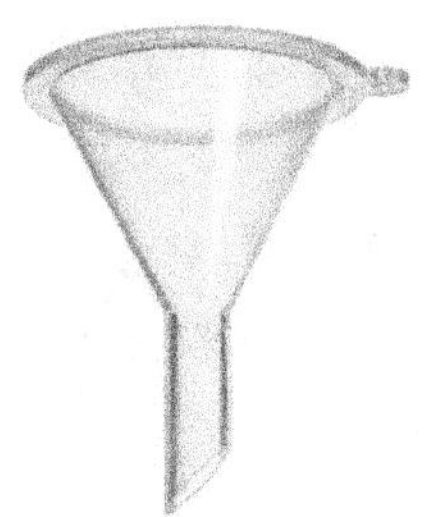

Bottle with pump dispenser

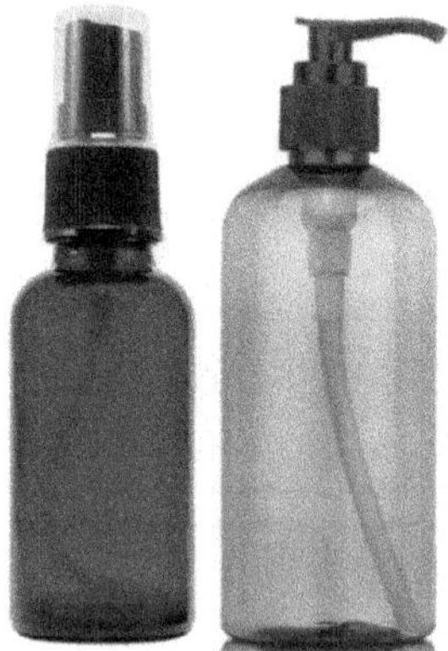

- <u>**Ingredients**</u>

Isopropyl, ethanol or rubbing alcohol (99 percent alcohol volume)

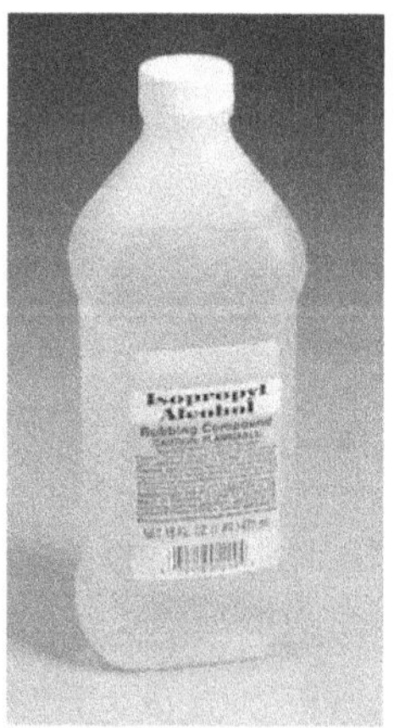

Rubbing alcohol, also called isopropyl alcohol, is a chemical substance diluted with water to make it effective in cleaning substances. Rubbing alcohol is an ideal chemical for disinfecting surfaces in the workplace or home. It is mainly used in hospitals to sterilize surgical tools, operation rooms, and sometimes to disinfect minor wounds or cuts. It is effective in killing pathogens that spread illness and infections.

Alcohol is the crucial ingredient that sanitizes and disinfects in hand sanitizer.

Active ingredients found in rubbing alcohol are:

Isopropyl alcohol - 91%

Aloe vera gel

Aloe vera is a thick, pointed, fleshy green leaves short-stemmed plant that stores water in its leaves.

Each leaf is filled with slimy tissue that stores water and makes the leaves thick.

The Aloe Vera "gel" is the slimy water-filled tissue. The leaves are packed with a gel-like material that contains many beneficial compounds.

There are different potent antioxidants compounds embedded in Aloe Vera gel, which can help prevent or decreases the spread of harmful bacteria.

You can buy an aloe vera gel from the store, or you can make your own

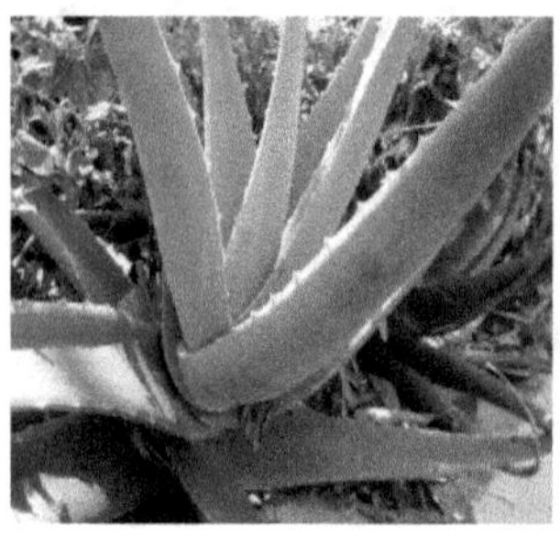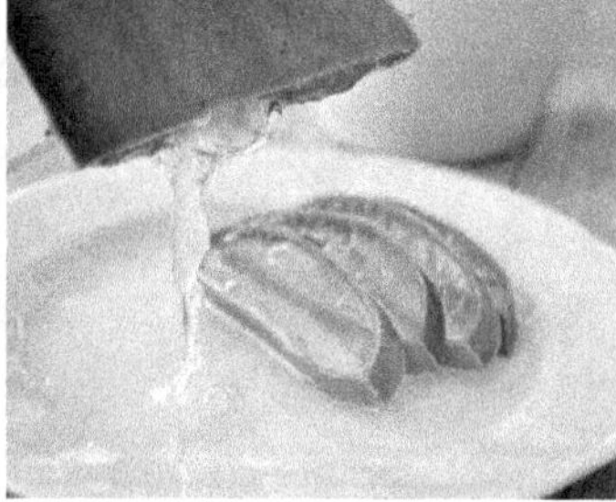

Essential oils

The essential oil is an oil extract from the seeds bark, stems roots, flowers, and other parts of plants. They are highly concentrated oil with strong aroma.it which gives plants their distinctive smells. The pure essential oil has a beautiful and powerful fragrant that is used for health care practices.

Essential oils are volatile aromatic compounds. This property makes it possible to change quickly from its solid or liquid state to a gas at room temperature.

The unique properties make essential oil ideal ingredient in the production of sanitizer (gel or spray)

Essential oil is known to have antibacterial, antimicrobial, antiviral, and antiseptic properties.

The essential oil is naturally safe and cost-effective.

8

They are different types of essential oils on the market, like rose oil, lavender oil, tea tree oil, and so much more. Make sure you get your essential oil from a good source.

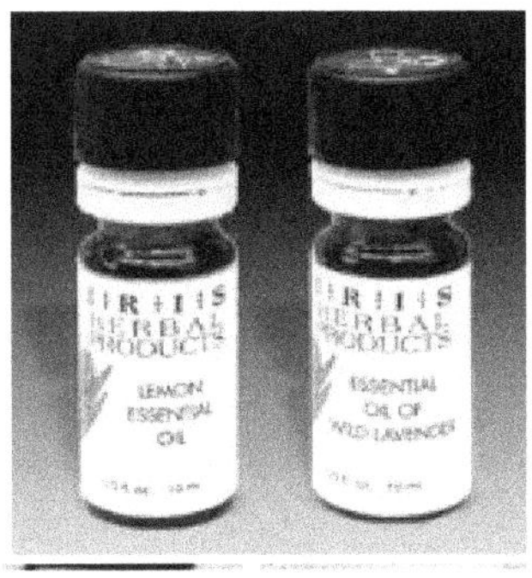

Glycerin

It helps the essential oils to disperse throughout the Alcohol, forms a protective layer, and moisturizes the skin.

It keeps the alcohol from drying fast from your body.

<u>Vitamin E</u>

One of the unique properties of vitamin E is that it moisturizes and helps to slow down rancidity.

<u>Carrier oil</u>

Carrier oil is a moisturizer and helps to dilute the essential oil safely. It also counterbalances the drying effect of witch hazel. Such as organic coconut oil, jojoba oil or sweet almond oil.

Chapter 3

Precaution to be taken when preparing alcohol-based Sanitizer

Always make sure you prepare hand sanitizers in a clean space

Ensure that the counter top or table is wiped with a dilute bleach solution.

Ensure your hand is washed thoroughly before preparing hand sanitizer

Use a clean bowl, spoon, whisk and bottle to avoid contamination.

Make sure the alcohol used for the hand sanitizer is the recommended one with alcohol content not less than 60%.

Combine and mix the ingredients thoroughly until you get a well-blended consistency.

Avoid touching the mixture with a bare hand until it is ready for use.

Use Nitrile gloves to prevent hand burn when making the hand sanitizer because Isopropyl alcohol is highly flammable.

Keep out of reach of children.

When ingested by accident, seek medical help immediately.

Main ingredients for most effective Alcohol-based hand sanitizer:

99% isopropyl alcohol (the hand sanitizer needs to contain at least 60% alcohol for it to be effective.

92% Aloe vera gel (act as a natural moisturizer)

Essential Oil (8 -10 drops of essential oils)

Mixing the ingredients:

While mixing the ingredients, you should maintain a 2:1 ratio of isopropyl alcohol to aloe vera gel.

If you add 2 oz of isopropyl alcohol, you will add 1 oz of aloe vera.

If you add 4 oz of isopropyl alcohol, you will add 2 oz of aloe vera and vice versa.

Follow the ratio and get the quantity you desire.

OR

2/3 cups of 99% isopropyl alcohol to 1/3 cup of 92% aloe vera gel.

Add drops of essential oil of your choice.

Allow the mixture to sit for 72 hours for the sanitizer to kill any bacteria introduce on the course of mixing as directed by W.H.O. (World Health Organization).

Chapter 4

Fast Gel Recipes with tea tree oil.

(Getting the ingredients direct from your cabinets, it does not require going out.).

Tea Tree oil sanitizer

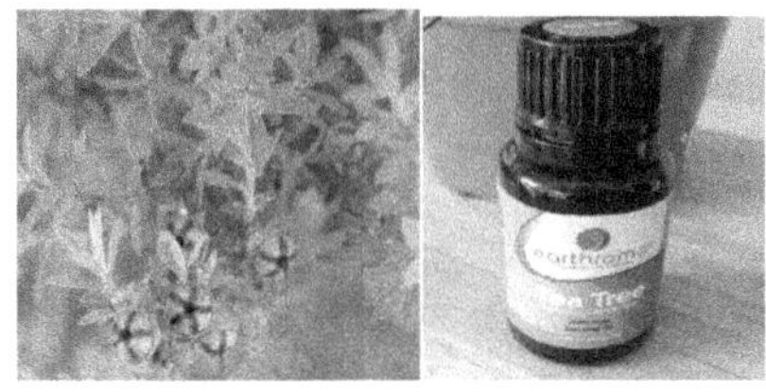

One of the active ingredients in tea tree oil is terpinen-4-ol which is effective in killing certain bacteria, fungi and viruses.

Ingredients

2/3 cups of Isopropyl alcohol

1/3 cups of Aloe vera gel

8 drops of Tea tree oil

Measure the quantities required, pour inside a bowl.

Combine isopropyl alcohol and aloe vera gel in a bowl and mix thoroughly.

Add drops of tea tree oil

Use the funnel to pour the liquid inside the bottle. Allow to sit for 72 hours before usage.

Final alcohol concentration:

Use 99% alcohol: to get 73.40%

Use 91% alcohol: to get 67.47%

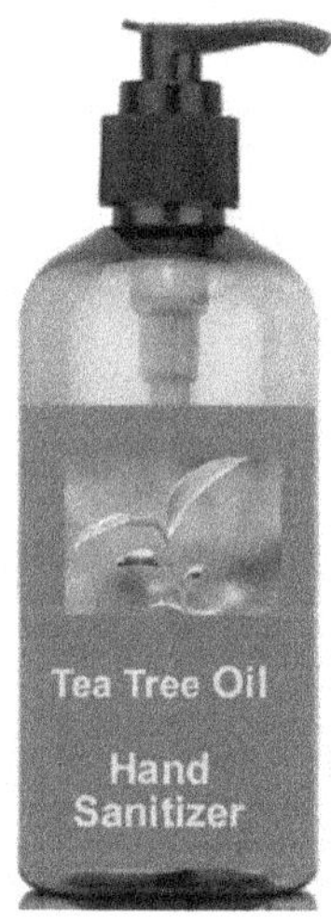

Lavender oil Sanitizer:

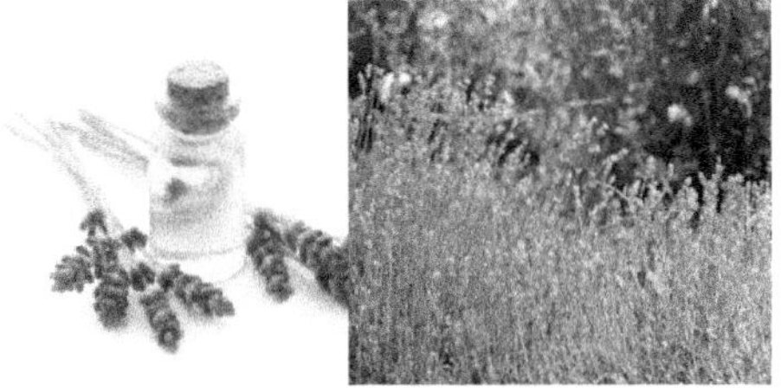

Lavender oil is an oil extracted from the Lavandula angustifolia Plant.

Its properties vary from antiseptic, antibacterial, antiviral, antimicrobial, and antifungal.

<u>Ingredients</u>

2/3 cups of Isopropyl alcohol

1/3 cups of Aloe vera gel

8 drops of Lavender oil

<u>Preparations</u>

Measure the quantities required, pour inside a bowl.

Combine isopropyl alcohol and aloe vera gel in a bowl and mix thoroughly.

Add drops of lavender oil

Use the funnel to pour the liquid inside the bottle. Allow to sit for 72 hours before usage.

Final alcohol concentration:

Use 99% alcohol: to get 73.40%

Use 91% alcohol: to get 67.47%

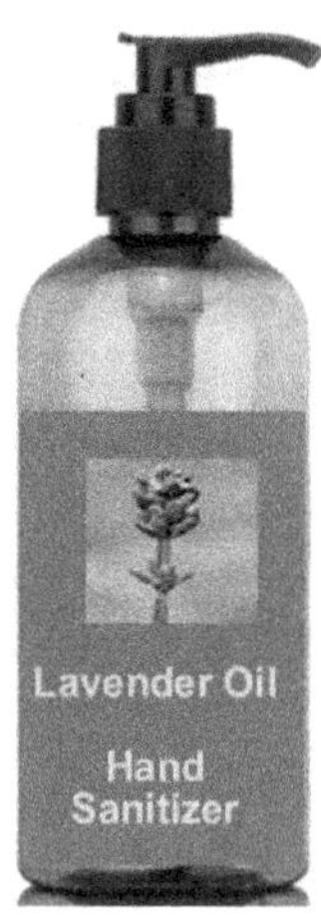

Geranium oil Sanitizer

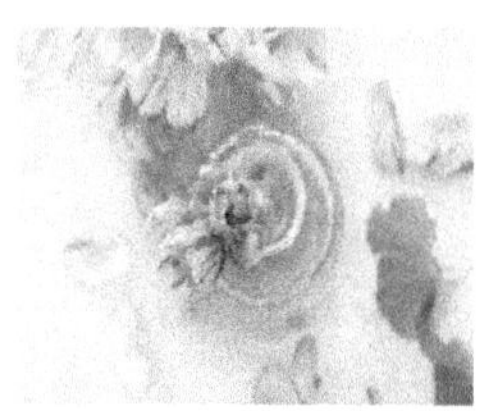

Geranium oil has Citronellol and Geraniol as an active ingredient that is responsible for antibacterial, antiviral, antifungal, and antiseptic.

16

Ingredients

2/3 cups of Isopropyl alcohol

1/3 cups of Aloe vera gel

8 drops of Geranium oil

Preparations

Measure the quantities required, pour inside a bowl.

Combine isopropyl alcohol and aloe vera gel in a bowl and mix thoroughly.

Add drops of geranium essential oil

Use the funnel to pour the liquid inside the bottle. Allow to sit for 72 hours before usage.

Final alcohol concentration:

Use 99% alcohol: to get 73.40%

Use 91% alcohol: to get 67.47%

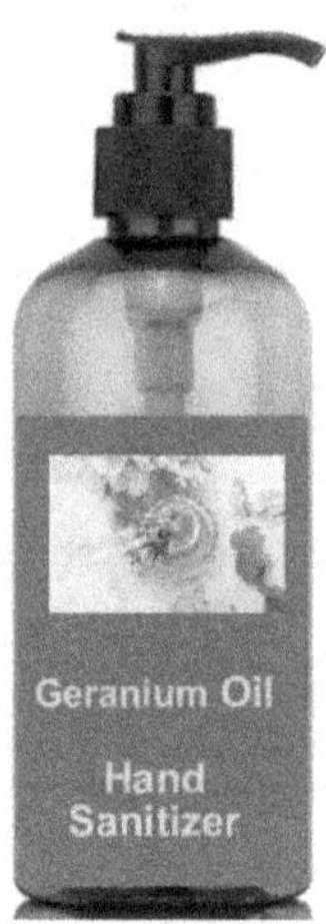

Lemon oil Sanitizer

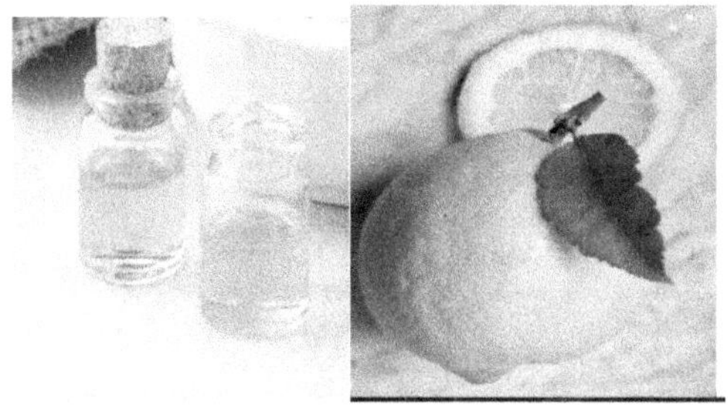

Lemon oil has antiseptic, antimicrobial, antifungal, and antiviral properties.

Use lemon oil with any carrier oil of your choice.

<u>Ingredients</u>

2/3 cups of Isopropyl alcohol

1/3 cups of Aloe vera gel

5 drops of lemon oil

5 drops of carrier oil

Preparations

Measure the quantities required, pour inside a bowl.

Combine isopropyl alcohol and aloe vera gel in a bowl and mix thoroughly.

Add drops of lemon and carrier oil

Use the funnel to pour the liquid inside the bottle. Allow to sit for 72 hours before usage.

Final alcohol concentration:

Use 99% alcohol: to get 73.40%

Use 91% alcohol: to get 67.47%

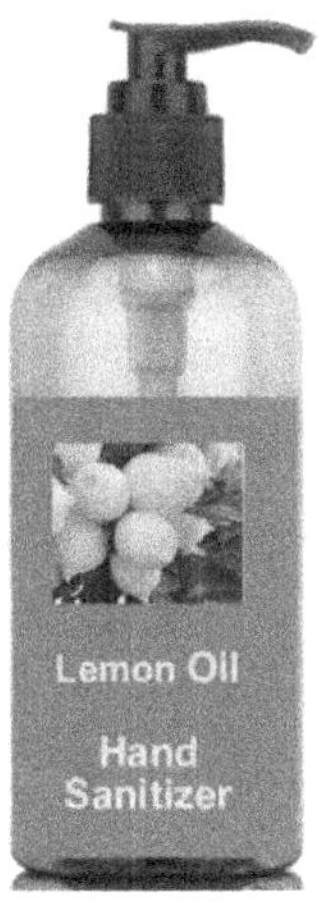

Sweet or wild orange oil Sanitizer

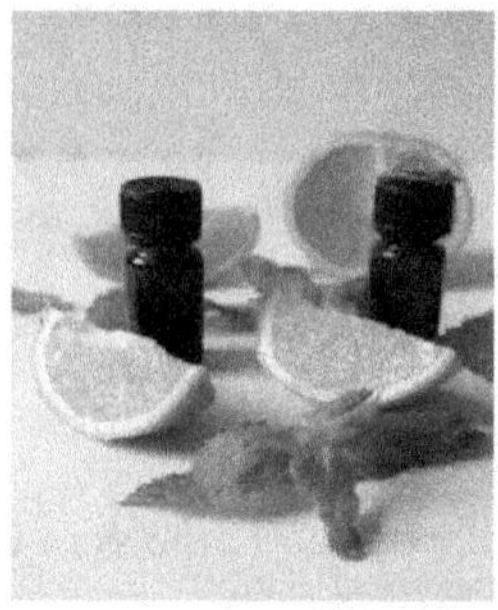

Sweet or wild orange has antiseptic antifungal, antiviral, and antibacterial properties.

Ingredients

2/3 cups of Isopropyl alcohol

1/3 cups of Aloe vera gel

8 drops of sweet orange oil

Preparation

Measure the quantities required, pour inside a bowl.

Combine isopropyl alcohol and aloe vera gel in a bowl and mix thoroughly.

Add drops of sweet orange oil

Use the funnel to pour the liquid inside the bottle. Allow to sit for 72 hours before usage

Final alcohol concentration:

Use 99% alcohol: to get 73.40%

Use 91% alcohol: to get 67.47%

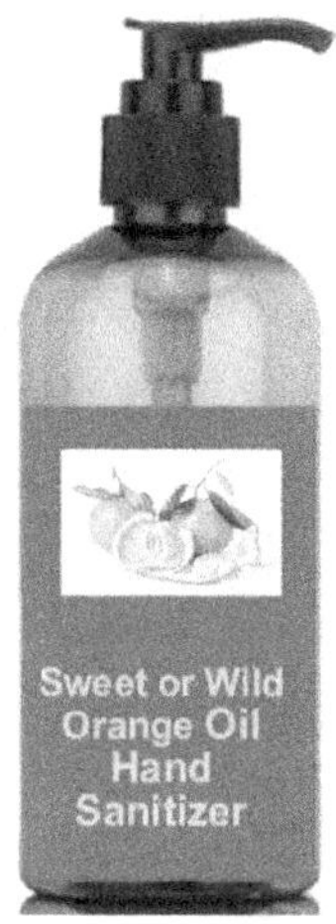

Eucalyptus + Tea tree oil Sanitizer

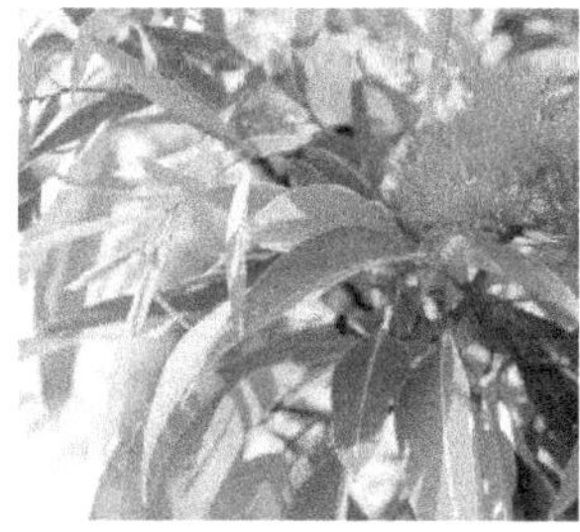

Eucalyptus oil has antibacterial, antiviral, antifungal, antimicrobial, and antiseptic properties.

Ingredients

2/3 cups of Isopropyl alcohol

1/3 cups of Aloe vera gel

4 drops of tea tree essential oil

6 drops of eucalyptus oil

Preparations

Measure the quantities required, pour inside a bowl.

Combine isopropyl alcohol and aloe vera gel in a bowl and mix thoroughly.

Add drops of eucalyptus and tea tree oil

Use the funnel to pour the liquid inside the bottle. Allow to sit for 72 hours before usage

Final alcohol concentration:

Use 91% alcohol: to get 67.47%

Use 99% alcohol: to get 73.40%

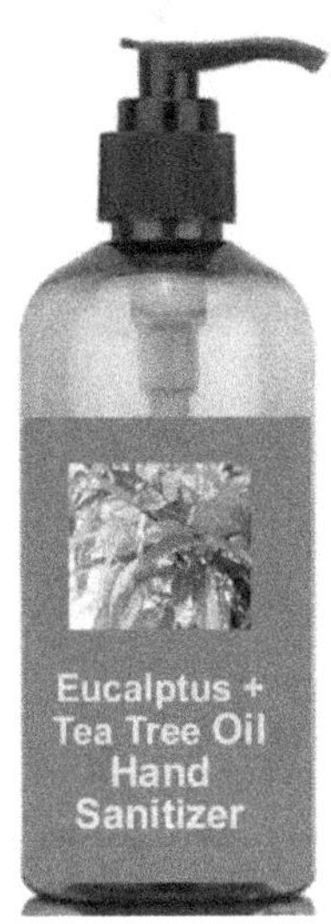

Rosemary oil Sanitizer

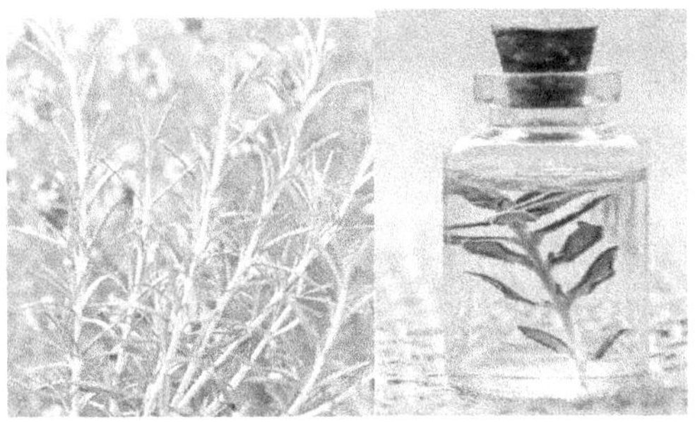

Rosemary oil has antiseptic, antifungal, antibacterial and antimicrobial properties.

<u>Ingredients</u>

2/3 cup of isopropyl alcohol (91% or 99%)

1/3 cup of aloe vera gel

6 drops of rosemary essential oil

3 drops of lemon essential oil

1 drop of tea tree essential oil

1/2 teaspoon of 98% glycerin

3 drops of vitamin E oil

<u>Preparation</u>

Measure the quantities required, pour inside a bowl.

Combine isopropyl alcohol, aloe vera gel, and glycerin in a bowl and mix thoroughly.

Add drops of Rosemary, lemon, tea tree, vitamin E and glycerin oil, stir until well blended.

Use the funnel to pour the liquid inside the bottle. Allow to sit for 72 hours before usage

Final alcohol concentration:

Use 91% alcohol: to get 67.47%

Use 99% alcohol: to get 73.40%

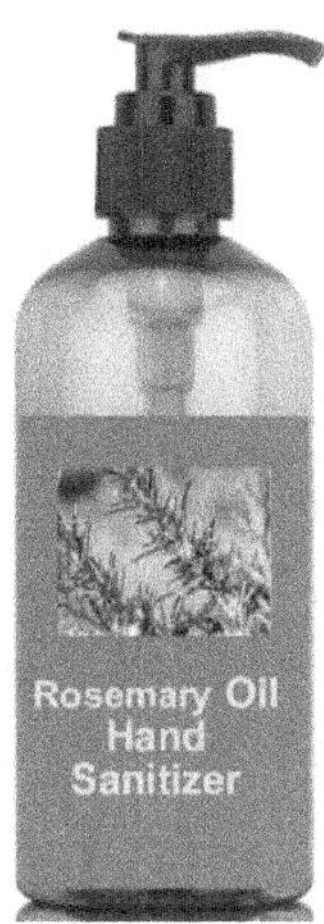

Cinnamon oil Sanitizer

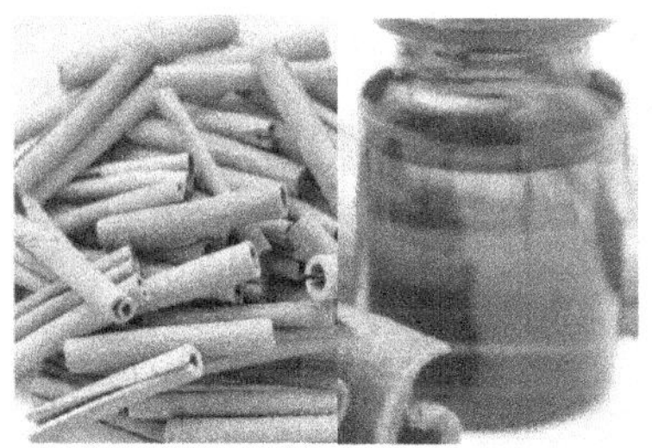

Cinnamon oil has antibacterial, antifungal, antiviral, antimicrobial, and antiseptic properties.

<u>Ingredients</u>

2/3 cup of isopropyl alcohol (91% or 99%)

1/3 cup of aloe vera gel

8 drops of Cinnamon essential oil

1 drop of tea tree essential oil

2 drops of vitamin E oil

Preparation

Measure the quantities required, pour inside a bowl.

Combine isopropyl alcohol and aloe vera gel in a bowl and mix thoroughly.

Add drops of Cinnamon, tea tree, and vitamin oil, stir until well blended.

Use the funnel to pour the liquid inside the bottle. Allow to sit for 72 hours before usage Final alcohol concentration:

Use 91% alcohol: to get 67.47%

Use 99% alcohol: to get 73.40%

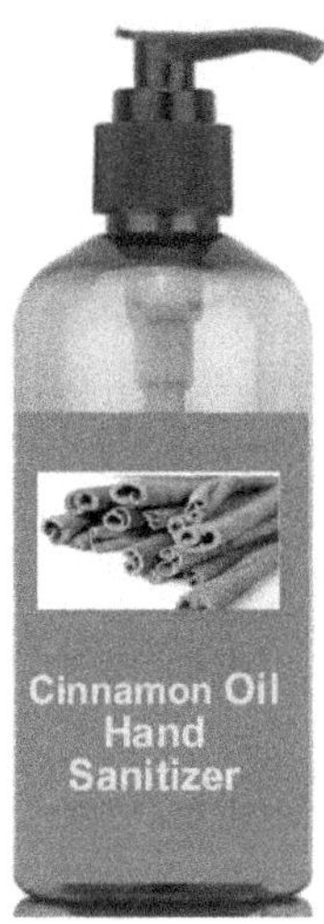

Clove oil Sanitizer

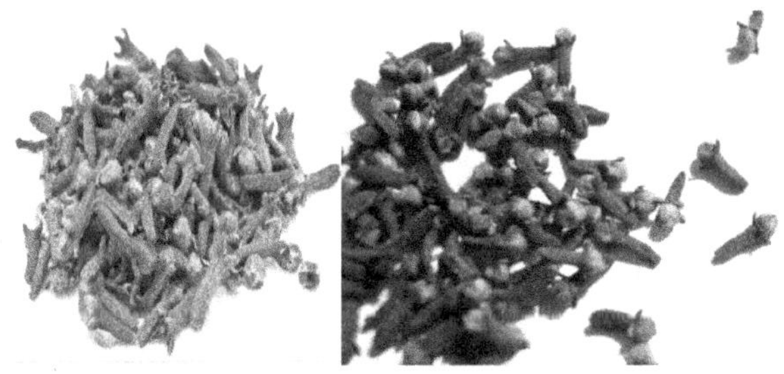

Clove essential oil is an oil derived from the clove tree; it has antiviral, antibacterial, antifungal, and antiseptic properties.

<u>Ingredients</u>

2/3 cup of isopropyl alcohol (91% or 99%)

1/3 cup of aloe vera gel

10 drops of clove essential oil

2 drops of vitamin E oil

Preparation

Measure the quantities required, pour inside a bowl.

Combine isopropyl alcohol and aloe vera gel in a bowl and mix thoroughly.

Add drops of Clove and vitamin E oil, stir until well blended.

Use the funnel to pour the liquid inside the bottle. Allow to sit for 72 hours before usage Final alcohol concentration:

Use 91% alcohol: to get 67.47%

Use 99% alcohol: to get 73.40%

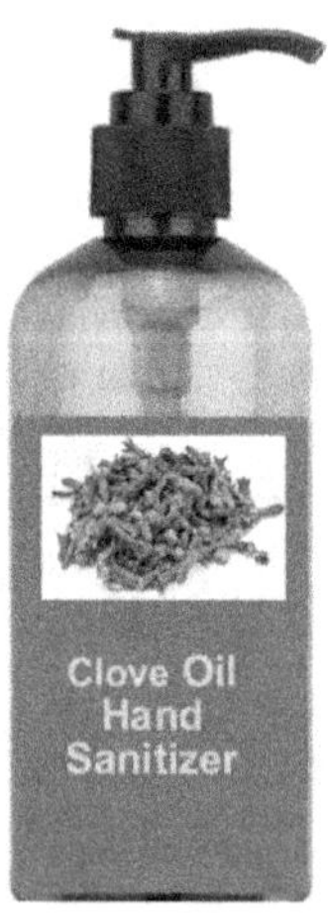

Thyme oil Sanitizer

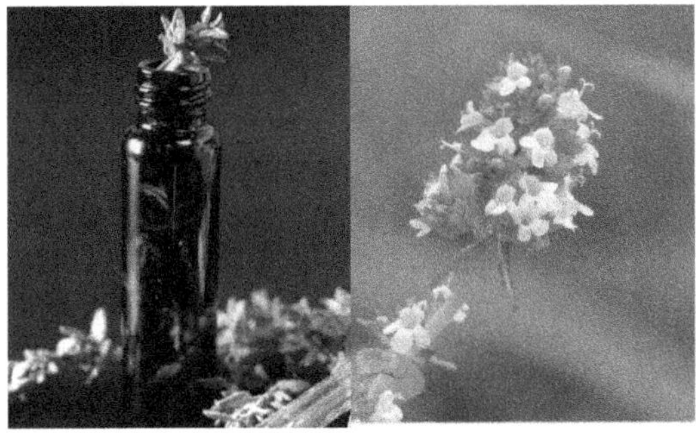

Thyme has antibacterial, antifungal, antimicrobial, antiseptic and antiviral properties

Ingredients

2/3 cup of isopropyl alcohol (91% or 99%)

1/3 cup of aloe vera gel

10 drops of thyme essential oil

2 drops of vitamin E oil

Preparation

Measure the quantities required, pour inside a bowl.

Combine isopropyl alcohol and aloe vera gel in a bowl and mix thoroughly.

Add drops of Thyme and vitamin E oil, stir until well blended.

Use the funnel to pour the liquid inside the bottle. Allow to sit for 72 hours before usage Final alcohol concentration:

Use 91% alcohol: to get 67.47%

Use 99% alcohol: to get 73.40%

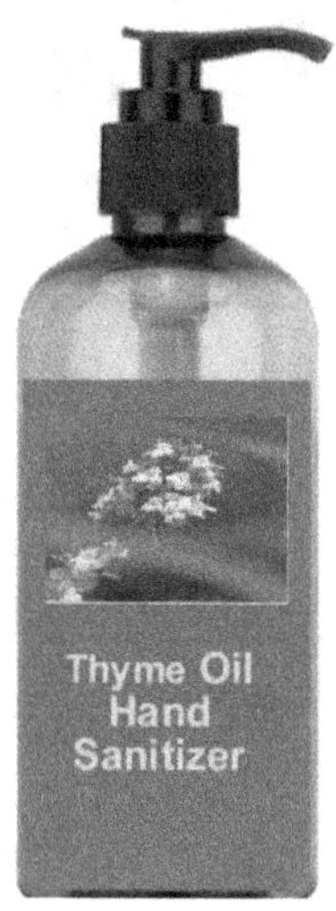

Peppermint oil sanitizer

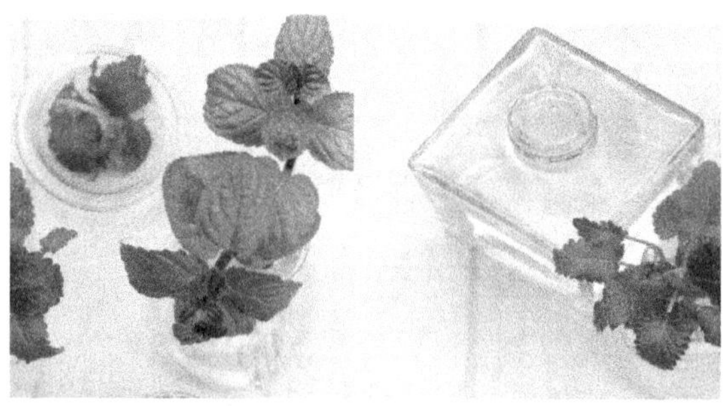

Peppermint oil has antiseptic, antiviral, and antibacterial properties.

Ingredients

2/3 cup isopropyl alcohol 99%

1/3 cup of aloe vera gel.

1 teaspoon glycerin

10 drops of peppermint essential oil

Preparation

Measure the quantities required, pour inside a bowl.

Combine isopropyl alcohol, aloe vera gel, and glycerin in a bowl and mix thoroughly.

Add drops of peppermint essential oil, stir until well blended.

Use the funnel to pour the liquid inside the bottle (dispenser). Allow to sit for 72 hours before usage

Final alcohol concentration:

Use 99% alcohol: to get 73.40%

Use 91% alcohol: to get 67.47%

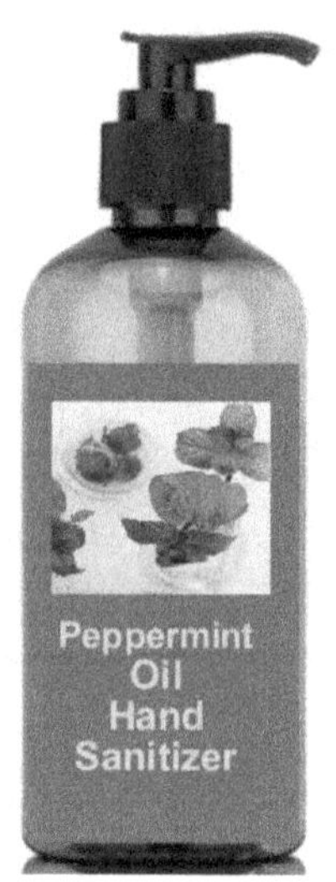

Peppermint
Oil
Hand
Sanitizer

Chapter 5

Special Combination Recipes

Recipes 1 (Thieves)

<u>Ingredients</u>

2/3 cup of isopropyl alcohol (91% or 99%)

1/3 cup of aloe vera gel

3 drops of Cinnamon Bark essential oil

3 drops of lemon essential oil

3 drops of eucalyptus oil

2 drops of peppermint essential oil

<u>Preparation</u>

Measure the quantities required, pour inside a bowl.

Combine isopropyl alcohol and aloe vera gel in a bowl and mix thoroughly.

Add drops of the essential oils mentioned above, stir until well blended.

Use the funnel to pour the liquid inside the bottle. Allow to sit for 72 hours before usage

Final alcohol concentration:

Use 99% alcohol: to get 73.40%

Use 91% alcohol: to get 67.47%

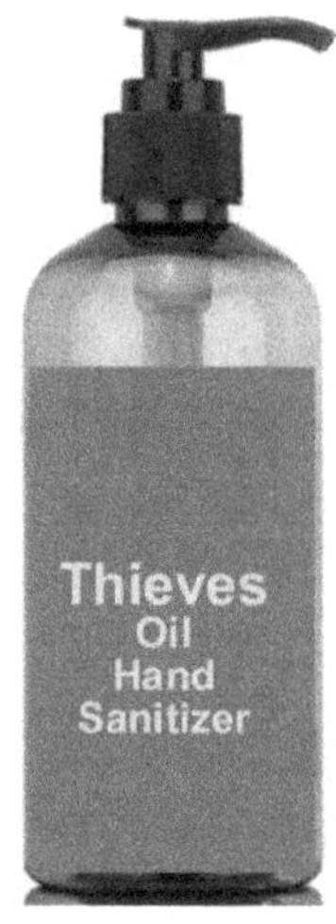

Recipes 2

Isopropyl alcohol, Aloe Vera, Thieves and Tea Tree

<u>Ingredients</u>

2/3 cup of isopropyl alcohol (91% or 99%)

1/3 cup of aloe vera gel

5 drops of Thieves essential oil

5 drops of Tea Tree oil

<u>Preparation</u>

Measure the quantities required, pour inside a bowl.

Combine isopropyl alcohol and aloe vera gel in a bowl and mix thoroughly.

Add drops of the essential oils mentioned above, stir until well blended.

Use the funnel to pour the liquid inside the bottle. Allow to sit for 72 hours before usage

Final alcohol concentration:

Use 99% alcohol: to get 73.40%

Use 91% alcohol: to get 67.47%

Recipe 3

Isopropyl Alcohol, Aloe Vera, Spearmint, Lavender, and Bergamot

Ingredients

2/3 cup of isopropyl alcohol (91% or 99%)

1/3 cup of aloe vera gel

4 drops of Spearmint essential oil

3 drops of Lavender oil

3 drops of Bergamont

<u>**Preparation**</u>

Measure the quantities required, pour inside a bowl.

Combine isopropyl alcohol and aloe vera gel in a bowl and mix thoroughly.

Add some drops of the essential oils mentioned above, stir until well blended.

Use the funnel to pour the liquid inside the bottle. Allow to sit for 72 hours before usage

Final alcohol concentration:

Use 99% alcohol: to get 73.40%

Use 91% alcohol: to get 67.47%

Recipes 4

Purification and lemon oil

<u>**Ingredients**</u>

2-ounce bottle with dispenser

2/3 cup of isopropyl alcohol (91% or 99%)

1/3 cup of aloe vera gel

5 drops of purification essential oil

3 drops of Lemon oil

I teaspoon of carrier oil

1 teaspoon of glycerin oil

Preparation

Measure the quantities required, pour inside a bowl.

Combine isopropyl alcohol, aloe vera gel, and glycerin oil in a bowl and mix thoroughly.

Add drops of the essential oils mentioned above, stir until well blended.

Use the funnel to pour the liquid inside the bottle. Allow to sit for 72 hours before usage

Final alcohol concentration:

Use 99% alcohol: to get 73.40%

Use 91% alcohol: to get 67.47%

Recipe 5

Germ Destroyer oil Sanitizer

Ingredients:

2/3 cup rubbing alcohol (91% or 99%)

1/2 tablespoons aloe vera gel

20 drops of Germ Destroyer Essential Oil.

<u>Preparations</u>

Mix the alcohol and aloe vera together until well blended, then add drops of essential oil. Miss gently and pour in a bottle.

Allow to sit for 72 hours before usage

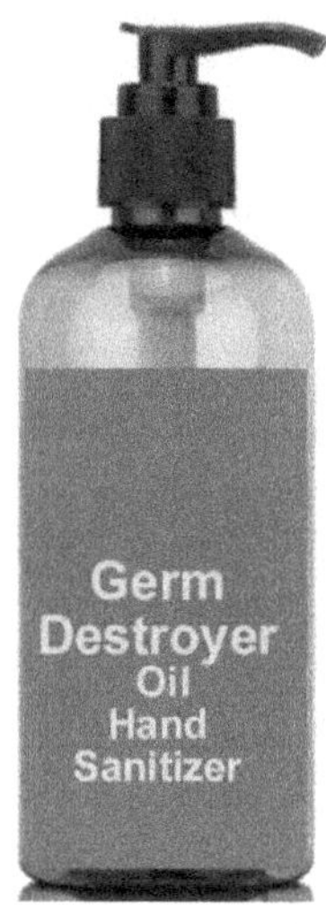

Fast (Spray) Recipe

<u>Ingredients</u>

12 oz of Isopropyl alcohol

2 teaspoons of Glycerol or glycerin (keep the alcohol from drying fast from your body)

1 tablespoon of Hydrogen peroxide

3 oz of Distilled water or boiled (later cooled) water.

Spray bottle

Remember the alcohol concentration in the mixture should not be less than 60%

Pour everything inside the spray bottle and shake for proper blending.

Use as a wipe.

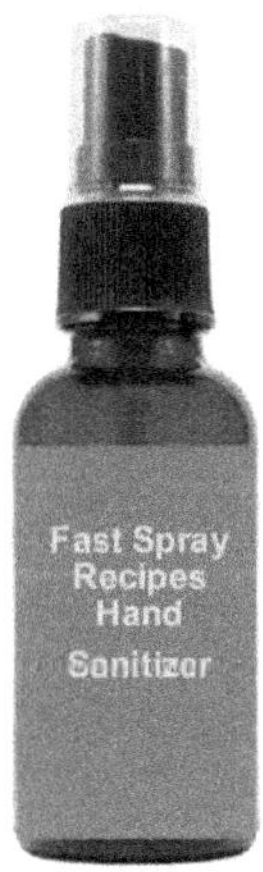

Combo Spray recipes

2/3 cup of Isopropyl alcohol, vitamin E oil, lemon oil, orange oil, tea tree oil, distilled water (or you can boil water and allow it to cool.)

<u>Ingredients</u>

2-ounce spray bottle
39

2/3 cup of isopropyl alcohol (91% or 99%)

3 tablespoons witch hazel with aloe vera.

4 drops of lemon essential oil

2 drops of vitamin E for soft hands

3 drops of orange essential oil

4 drops of tea tree essential oil

I teaspoon of carrier oil

1/2 teaspoon of glycerin oil

Preparations

Measure the quantities of the ingredients required, pour inside a spray bottle. Tightly place the sprayer and shake for about 20- 25 seconds to combine.

Open the bottle and fill with water to the brim.

Replace the cap and shake well again for about 20-25 seconds.

Allow to sit for 72 hours before usage

Final alcohol concentration:

Use 99% alcohol: to get 73.40%

Use 91% alcohol: to get 67.47%

Shake the bottle vigorously to reincorporate the essential oils, then spray a generous amount on your hands

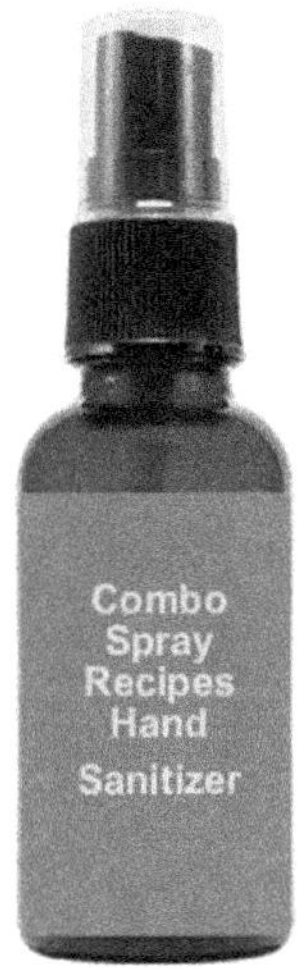

Chapter 6

Guidelines to follow/ frequently asked questions

1. Always use isopropyl alcohol (91% or 99%)

   In a situation where it is not available, you can use 3/4 cup of 190 proof grain (ethyl) alcohols together with 1/4 of aloe vera gel.

The ratio of alcohol to aloe vera depends on the % content of alcohol you are using.

<u>Illustration</u>

If you're using 99% Isopropyl rubbing alcohol, you'll need a different quantity of aloe vera compared to when you are using 70% alcohol.

Follow the quick guidelines below?

Sample 1

99% Isopropyl or Rubbing Alcohol:

2 parts alcohol = 2/3 cup of alcohol

1 part aloe vera gel = 1/3 cup of aloe vera gel

Sample 2

70% Isopropyl or Rubbing Alcohol:

9 parts alcohol = 90ml or 3 ounces of alcohol

1 part aloe vera gel = 10ml or 2 teaspoons

Sample 3

91% Isopropyl or Rubbing Alcohol.

3 parts alcohol = 3/4 cup alcohol

4 part aloe vera gel = 1/4 cup aloe vera gel

NOTE: Don't use other types of alcohol (such as methanol and butanol) because they're toxic.

2.   My Consistency is too thick

If you observed that your homemade hand sanitizer is too thick and won't enter into a bottle.

You are advised to add more rubbing alcohol until you get a pourable consistency.

3.   How long does homemade sanitizer last?

The shelf life depends on the ingredients used. If you use fresh aloe vera gel, make sure you keep the solution in the fridge and use within 2 weeks.

Hand sanitizer lasts for about a year when you use all shelf-stable ingredients (without water). For example,

Store-bought aloe vera gel   2 years

Glycerin   4-6 years

Witch hazel   4-5 years

Note: Diluting the ingredients with alcohol and essentials oil has no or little effect on the shelf life of the sanitizer.

4. <u>Storage?</u>

Hand sanitizer is not supposed to be kept for so long, but if you decided otherwise or you have produced much, that will last for long. I advise storing it in the refrigerator to be safe.

5. <u>Where can I get a bottle for my hand sanitizer?</u>

You can use an old cosmetics bottle, or you can buy 2-ounce pump bottles from your local store.

6. <u>Can I use other ingredients?</u>

To get an effective hand sanitizer that kills germs, use an only alcohol-based recipe

7. <u>What is the effect of cold-pressed lemon essential oil to the body?</u>

A cold-pressed lemon essential oil should be diluted with carrier oil at a rate of 12 drops of lemon oil to 1 ounce of carrier oil. Or 2-3 drops of lemon essential oil to 1 teaspoon of carrier and 1/2 teaspoon of glycerin oil.

This dilution helps to stop a phototoxic skin reaction when tropically exposed to the sun.

45

www.ingramcontent.com/pod-product-compliance
Lightning Source LLC
Chambersburg PA
CBHW050749250726
48662CB00005B/2108